H₂O Workouts®

Half Noodle

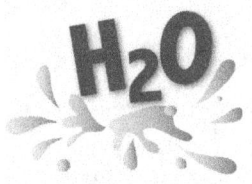

Francine Milford, LMT

H2OWorkouts® Half Noodle by Francine Milford, LMT
Copyright© 2012 Francine Milford, LMT

Photographs by Paul, Larry and Francine Milford

ID: 978-1-105-88391-0

Caution
The techniques, ideas, and suggestions presented in this book are not intended as a substitute for proper medical advice. Any application of the techniques, ideas, and suggestions in this book is at the reader's sole discretion and risk.

Please consult your health care provider before beginning this or any other exercise program.

www.H2Oworkouts.com

Fitness for the Next Generation

As more people are recognizing the need to live healthier and better lives, they have begun to set goals on how they will achieve and maintain a healthy body through proper nutrition and balanced work schedules.

Before long, the entire face of a typical aerobic class was changed as millions of people attempted to find a way to add exercise into their daily lives. Classes ranged in levels from easy senior workouts and classes for pregnant women to the high paced, high intensity Boot Camp classes.

Soon, many people were experiencing injuries from pushing their bodies too long and too far. When people are impatient to see results, they tend to exercise for long hours in a short period of time. Overuse injuries are one of the most common injuries found in the fitness industry.

Now most facilities offer Tai Chi, Qigong, Yoga and Pilates for people who want a good workout without the stress and strain of strenuous exercise.

The Great Equalizer

I call the water environment, the Great Equalizer. When I have taught water aerobic classes I would have ladies enter the water on crutches and even one came to class in a wheelchair. Once in the water, you could not tell the ladies apart. In the water environment, everyone is equal and everyone can receive a workout that is right for them and their fitness level.

In this book I will be sure to list exercises in **LEVELS**. If you are a beginner, then please stick to **Level One** exercises. As your body becomes familiar with the moves and becomes stronger, then move on up to **Level Two** and **Level Three**.

Principles of Water Exercise

The water environment offers two important natural occurring effects to the water routine: buoyancy and resistance. Buoyancy is the property of being able to float. Buoyancy is also the power of a liquid to keep objects afloat; in this case, that object is you.

It is the natural ability of water to act as a cushion and in so doing, it protects you joints from injury, strain and re-injury. Many rehabilitation centers use the water environment in their treatment sessions.

While in the water environment, people can perform exercises they otherwise could not on land. Among these exercises are jumps, leaps, jumping jacks and pivots. Amazingly enough, the ability of water to be buoyant also allows water to provide resistance to water aerobics. Through changing direction, adding speed, or using longer levers, the water can provide a complete and thorough workout.

The water environment can become a natural total body workout. The more you put into your workout, the more you will receive from it. The faster you move, the harder the exercise becomes.

Water aerobics is also the perfect environment for those who are overweight or suffer from physical injuries. When you stand in water that is chest deep, you weigh only 10% of your normal body weight.

The water environment is also the great place to practice your golf or tennis swing. Even dancers and weight trainers can use the resistance in the water to build up muscles in a safe way.

Tips for a Safe Workout

Do's and Dont's
- Do wear aqua shoes or aqua socks
- Do keep head in alignment of the spine.
- Do exercise in water that is of correct depth for you.
- Do relax and breathe slowly and deeply.
- Drink plenty of water before, during, and after exercising.
- Consult with your doctor before you begin exercising.
- Work at your own fitness level.
- Stop exercising if you feel faint, dizzy, nausea, or shortness of breath.
- Don't smoke or drink alcohol while exercising.
- Don't make fast, uncontrolled movements of the head or trunk in any direction.
- Don't use extreme range of motion.
- Don't use quick, jerky movement.
- Don't exercise with food or gum in your mouth.
- If you feel tired-stop
- For safety, there should be a lifeguard on duty during your workout or invite a friend to exercise with you.
- Never drink alcohol before, during, or immediately after a water workout.
- Perform your exercises in water that is chest high.
- Wait at least 1-3 hours after eating before working out
- When you enter the water that is cool, be sure to beginning walking, jogging, or bouncing right away to get your circulation moving.
- Always begin exercising slowly and then working up to more strenuous, energetic moves.
- Remember-Have fun!

Workout in Water

Warm-ups

As in any exercise program, it is important to prepare the body for the work that you are planning to put it through. We call this preparation, the Warm-Up.

In the Warm-Up you will increase the flow of blood to each and every muscle of the body. In this way, you will greatly reduce the risk of injury.

Warm-up exercises are usually gentle and slow activities that normally last 5 to 15 minutes. During this phase all the muscles and joints should be put through simple movements beginning with small range of motions and then increasing to larger, or full, range of motion.

In a typical land aerobic or workout class, we begin simply with marching in placing. The same holds true for water aerobics. In this chapter we will include several muscle groups that you will need to be sure you warm-up before beginning a water aerobics class. For some, this may be all the exercise that you can do in one day and if so, that is perfectly okay. What is important is move and stretch your body as often as you can throughout the day to keep it limber and lubricated.

When I received my certification in Aquatic Exercise, we practiced many types of water walking. Following a 3 to 5 minute warm-up exercise (such as marching in place) you could do some of the following walking exercises for the next 20-45 minutes:

- Walk forward and backwards
- Walk to the right and Walk to the left
- Walk in a big clockwise circle, then walk in a big counter-clockwise circle
- Walk on your toes

- Walk on your heels
- Walk like a crab sideways bouncing from flat feet with knees bent and open to the sides of your body.
- Walk forward and backward punching the water.
- Walk three steps and hop for one step.
- Do the Congo step in the water.
- Do the Bunny hop in the water.
- Do the Electric Slide in the water.
- Do your favorite Western Two Step in the water.
- Alternate between fast and slow walking to add intensity.
- Do the Soldier Walk, otherwise known on Goose Stepping
- Do Karate Kicks
- Walk doing knee lifts forward and front leg lift backwards
- Do Pendulum Swings with your legs side to side
- Do the Rocking Horse forward and backwards and change legs.
- Do Hamstring Curls forward and backwards.
- When stretching muscles in the warm-up phase it would be good if you could hold each stretch for at least 10 seconds (30 seconds is optimal).

Stretching

When performing the warm-up exercises and stretches, you should be able to feel slight warmth within your body. This is good and signals that you are preparing your body for the more vigorous workout that is to follow. The muscles that are stretched during the warm-up phase are the muscles that will be worked through the aerobic phase.

The Toe and Ankle Warm-ups

Some warm-up exercises and stretches can be performed inside, or at poolside, before you ever enter the water. If you find it difficult to spend more than 20 minutes in the water, then performing the warm-up stretches before entering the water may be a good idea. Remember, do the best that you can but don't push your body beyond its physical limitation and most of all – Have Fun!

Toes and Ankles

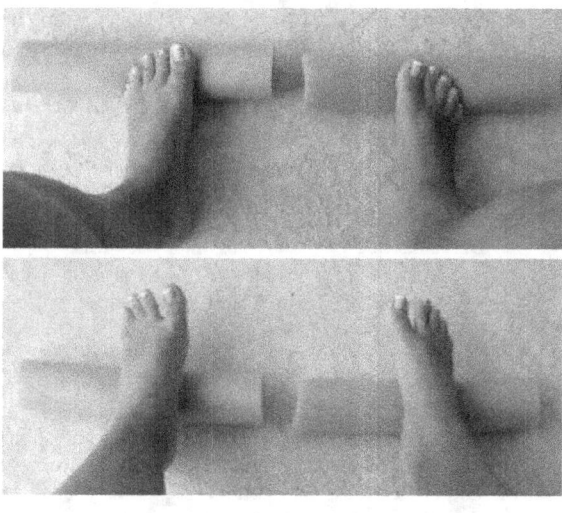

To Do: Roll your feet toes to heel and back again over the pool noodle. Do this exercise for eight repetitions.

Toes and Ankles

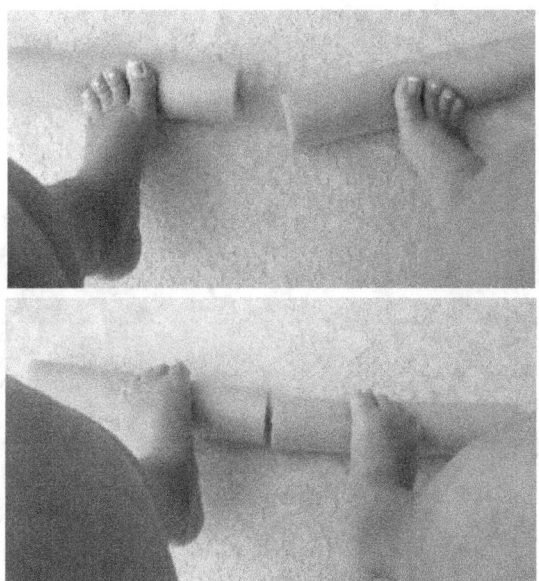

To Do: Stretch your toes up towards you, hold and count for 10 seconds. Release your toes down and press them into the noodle and hold that press for 10 seconds. Repeat this series for a total of eight repetitions.

Toes and Ankles

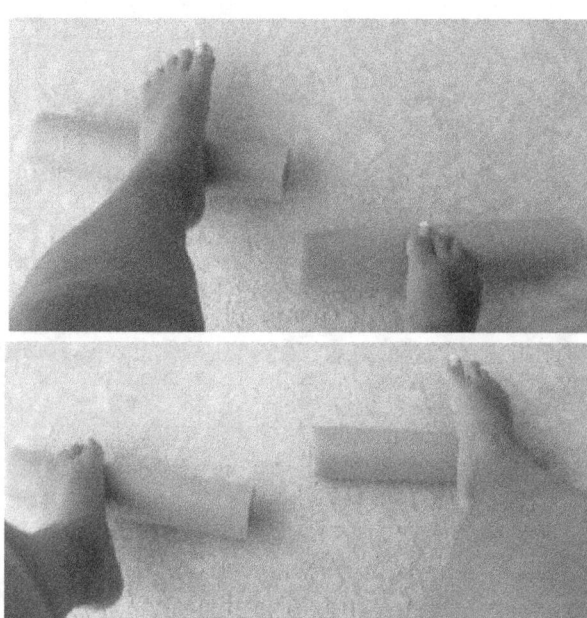

To Do: Between with your feet on the inside of the noodle and start rolling your feet back and forth moving to the outside of the noodle. Roll back in towards the center and out again for a total of eight repetitions.

Warm-ups for the Neck

Like the warm-ups for the toes and ankles, warm-ups for the neck can be performed on land before you enter the water environment. Do not push these stretches beyond what your physical capabilities are. Stretches should not be painful. If they are, stop immediately and consult with your primary health care provider.

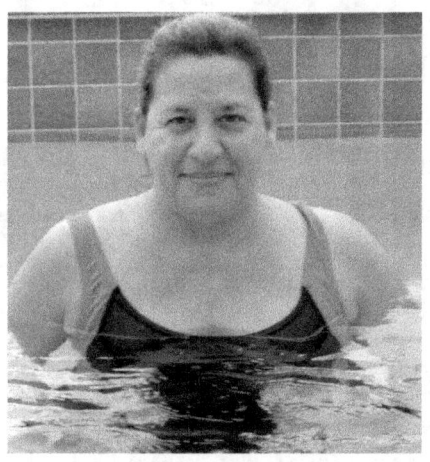

Starting Position

The starting point for the neck exercises will begin with the head in a neutral position as is shown in the diagram above, on the left. Keep you gaze in front of you at a slight angle downward. Be sure to breathe normally.

Neck Warm-ups

Neck

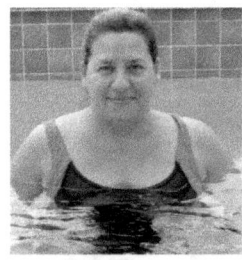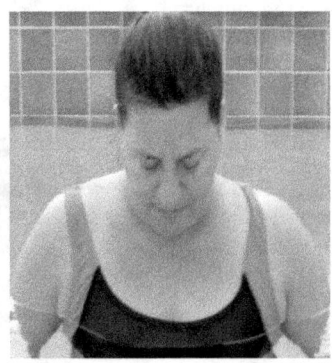

To Do: With your head in the starting position take a nice deep slow breath in. As you exhale, slowly allow your head to fall forward touching your chin to your chest (note: if you cannot touch your chin to your chest, this is alright, don't force the movement.)

Now, slowly inhale and begin to return your head to the starting position. Repeat this exercise for a total of eight repetitions.

Neck

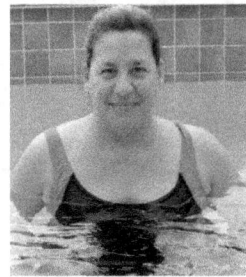
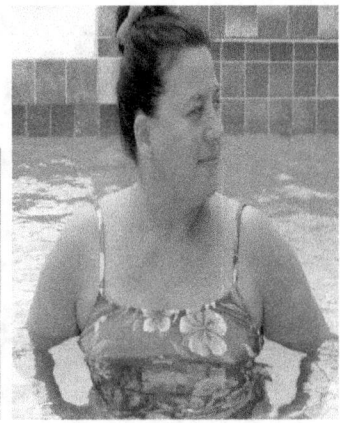

To Do: With your head in the starting position take a nice deep slow breath in. As you exhale, slowly turn your head to left aligning your chin to over your left shoulder (note: if you cannot align your chin to over your shoulder, this is alright, don't force the movement.)

Now, slowly inhale and as you exhale, begin to return your head to the starting position. With your head in the starting position take a nice deep slow breath in. As you exhale, slowly turn your head to right aligning your chin to over your right shoulder (note: if you cannot align your chin to over your shoulder, this is alright, don't force the movement.) Repeat this exercise for a total of eight repetitions.

Neck

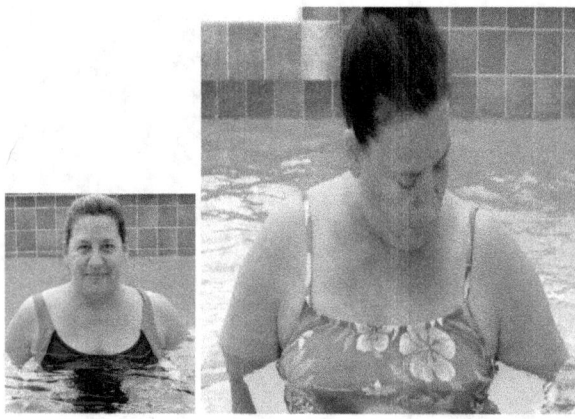

To Do: With your head in the starting position take a nice deep slow breath in. As you exhale, slowly allow your chin to drop to the left to a point that is located half way between the center of your chest and your left shoulder (note: if you cannot touch your chin to your chest, this is alright, don't force the movement.) Now, slowly inhale and as you exhale, begin to return your head to the starting position.

With your head in the starting position take a nice deep slow breath in. As you exhale, slowly allow your chin to drop to the right to a point that is located half way between the center of your chest and your right shoulder. Repeat this exercise for a total of eight repetitions.

Neck

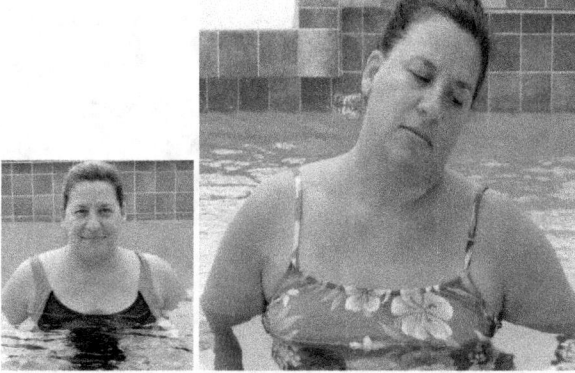

To Do: With your head in the starting position take a nice deep slow breath in. As you exhale, slowly allow your left ear to drop to your left shoulder (note: if you cannot touch your ear to your shoulder, this is alright, don't force the movement.)

Now, slowly inhale and as you exhale, begin to return your head to the starting position.

With your head in the starting position take a nice deep slow breath in. As you exhale, slowly allow your right ear to drop to your right shoulder (note: if you cannot touch your ear to your shoulder, this is alright, don't force the movement.)

Repeat this exercise for a total of eight repetitions.

Neck

Head Rolls

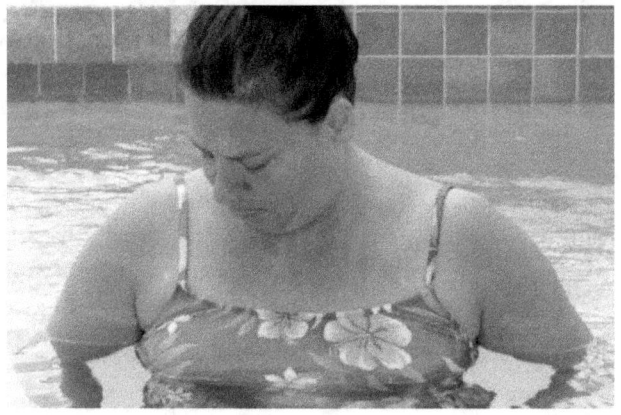

To Do: Imagine that your nose is like the hands of wall clock. The numbers of the wall clock are right in front of your face. Take a nice deep slow breath in and as you slowly exhale you will begin with your nose in the twelve o'clock position. Moving clockwise outline the numbers of the clock from 3, to 6, to 9, and ending back at the top at the number 12 position. Repeat for eight repetitions.

Now, repeat the above exercise, this time moving counter clockwise beginning at the 12 position moving down to the 9, 6, 3, and back to the top 12 position. Repeat for eight repetitions.

Warm-up for the Shoulders

Shoulders

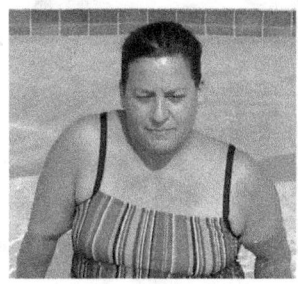 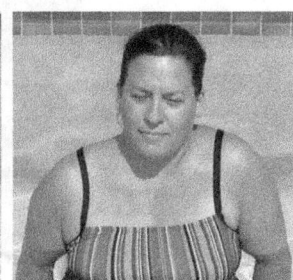

To Do: Begin by planting both feet flat on the bottom of the pool. Bend your knees slightly and arms down at your sides. Now, standing perfectly straight, inhale and bring your right shoulder up to your right ear and hold. As you exhale release the shoulder back down to starting position. Remember-do NOT bring your ear down to meet the shoulder. This is very important. Repeat for a total of 8 repetitions. Now, inhale and bring your left shoulder up to your left ear and hold. As you exhale, relax and return to the starting position. Repeat for a total of 8 repetitions.

Alternating Shoulders: Inhale and bring your right shoulder up to your right ear and hold. Exhale and relax the shoulder back to the starting position. Inhale and bring your left shoulder up to your left ear and hold. Exhale and relax the shoulder back to the starting position. Repeat for a total of 16 repetitions.

Shoulders – Shrugs

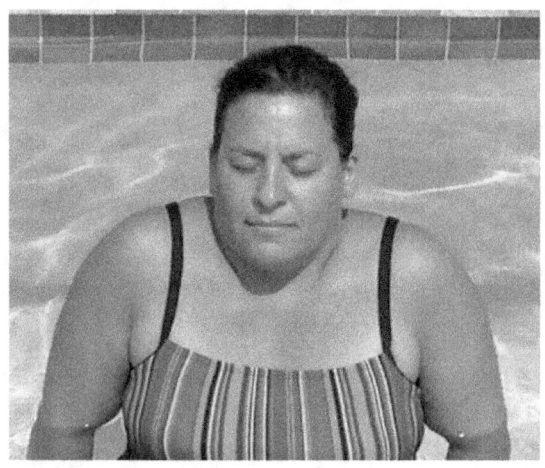

To Do: Inhale and bring both of your shoulders up to your ears and hold for a few seconds. As you exhale, allow both shoulders to relax and return to the starting position. Continue for a total of 16 repetitions. This is a great exercise to do throughout the day to reduce stress.

Shoulders – Circles

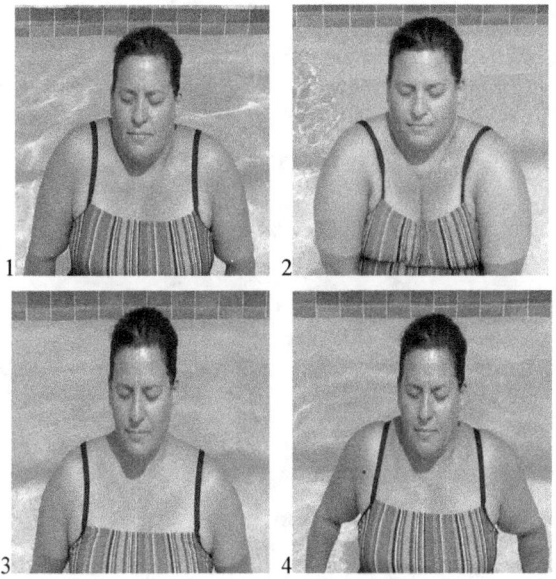

To Do: Inhale and bring both shoulders up to your ears (1) and as you exhale allow the shoulders to push forward (2), then down (3), then back behind you (4) forming a circle. As you inhale again pull the shoulders back up to your ears and repeat the circle of exhaling and allowing the shoulders to drop to the front, down to the sides and to the back before returning up to the ears again. Repeat 8 x's. When finished, repeat this exercise making circles in the opposite direction. Repeat for a total of eight repetitions.

Warm-up for the Wrists

If you have any wrist problems or injuries---please consult your health care provider before beginning these exercises.

Wrist Starting Position

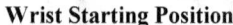

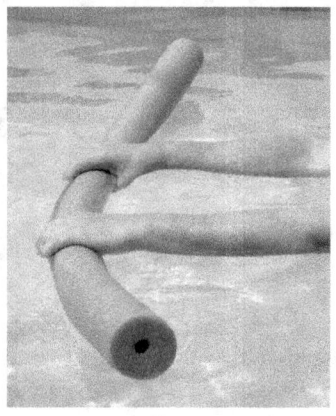

Starting Position: Begin the following exercises in the starting position as shown in the picture above. Plant both of your feet firmly on the bottom of the pool with knees slightly bent. Be sure that your knees are shoulder width apart. Extend both of your arms straight out in front of your body with fingers pointing away from your body. Keep your arms straight but do not lock your elbows. Keep a soft, but firm grip on the pool noodle. This is the starting position.

Wrist

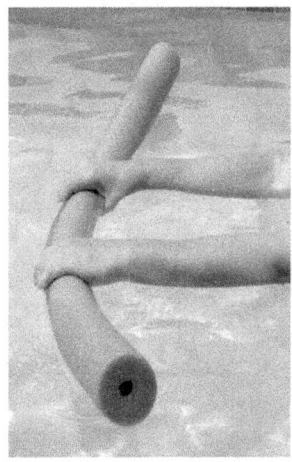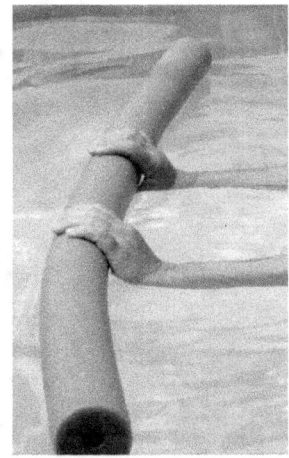

To Do: Take a nice slow, deep breath and at the same time, lift the fingers of both of your hands towards you while keeping the heel of your hand pushing away from your body, hold the stretch for a few seconds.

As you slowly exhale, lower your fingers back to the starting position as shown in the picture above, on the left.

Repeat for a total of eight repetitions.

Wrists

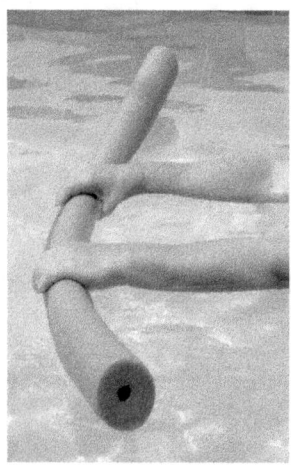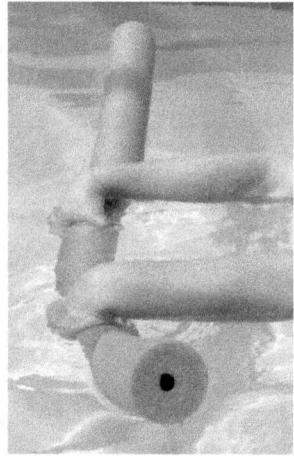

To Do: Extend both of your arms straight out in front of your body. Do not lock your elbows. If this is uncomfortable, just relax your arms and do the best that you can. Take a nice slow, deep breath and at the same time, point the fingers of both of your hands down towards the bottom of the pool, while keeping your arms extended away from your body, hold the stretch for a few seconds.

As you slowly exhale, raise your fingers back to the starting position as shown in the picture above, on the left. Repeat for a total of eight repetitions.

Finger Exercises

Starting Position

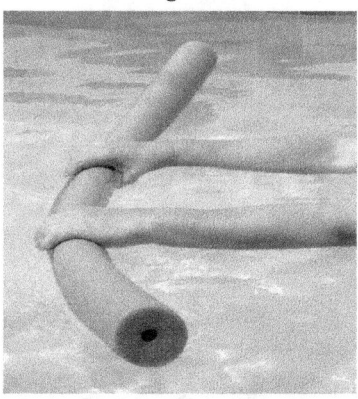

To Do: To perform the following finger exercises you will need to begin in the starting position as shown below. You will place you hands on the pool noodle at about shoulder width apart. Keep your knees bent and breathe regularly. Start with the index finger of both of your hands and apply slight pressure to the pool noodle, hold and count to eight, then release the pressure. Continue to press, hold and count, and release for a total of eight repetitions.

Repeat the entire process using your middle finger, the ring finger and ending with the little pinkie finger. If you feel uncomfortable or experience any pain, stop immediately.

Index Finger

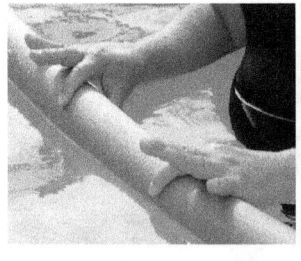

Middle Finger

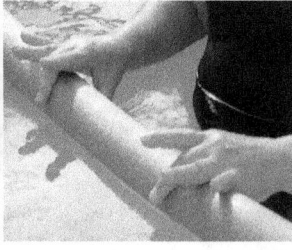

Ring Finger

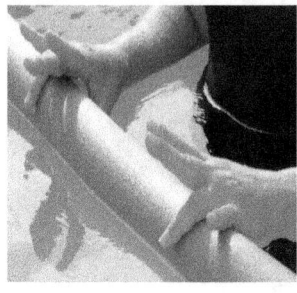

Pinkie

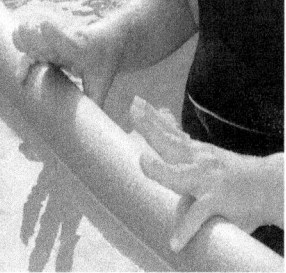

Arms and Shoulders

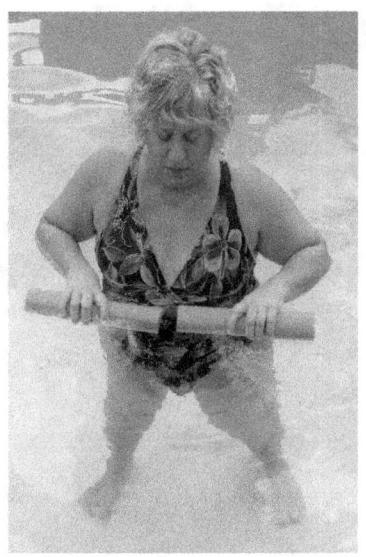

Starting Position

To Do: Place your hands on the center of the half noodle.
Keep your feet flat on the bottom of the pool with your knees
slightly bent.

Arms and Shoulders

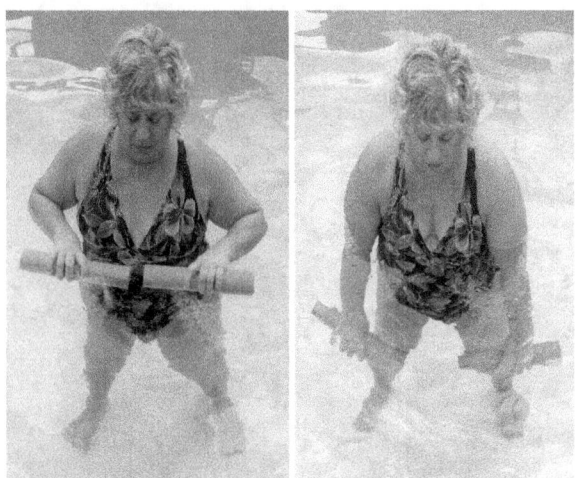

To Do: Place your hands on the center of the half noodle. Keep your feet flat on the bottom of the pool with your knees slightly bent. Inhale, and as you exhale push the noodles straight down into the water towards the bottom of the pool.

Inhale and as you exhale, bring the noodle back to your chest. Repeat for a total of at least eight repetitions.

Chest

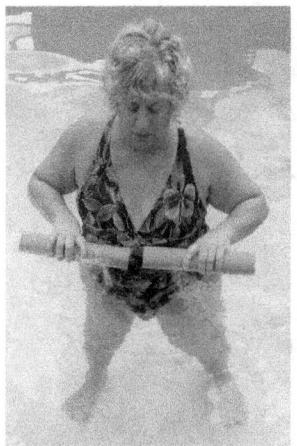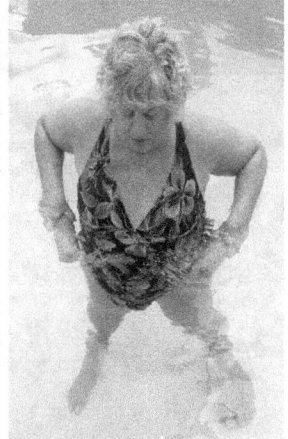

To Do: Place your hands on the center of the half noodle. Keep your feet flat on the bottom of the pool with your knees slightly bent. Inhale, and as you exhale bring the pool noodle toward the sides of your body.

Inhale and as you exhale, bring the noodle back to the front of your chest. Repeat for a total of at least eight repetitions.

Arms and Shoulders

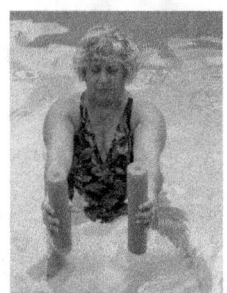

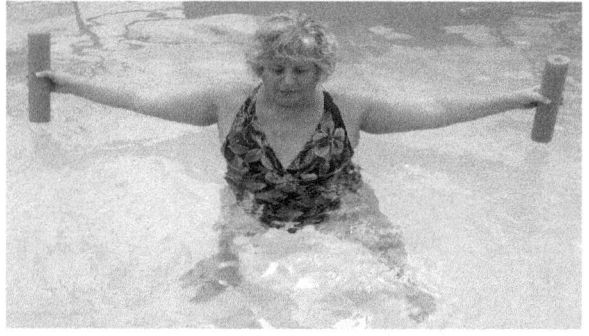

To Do: Place your hands on the center of the half noodle. Keep your feet flat on the bottom of the pool with your knees slightly bent. Inhale, and as you exhale bring the pool noodle toward the sides of your body. (Keep the noodle above the water). Inhale and as you exhale, bring the noodle back to the front of your chest. Repeat for a total of at least eight repetitions.

Arms and Shoulders

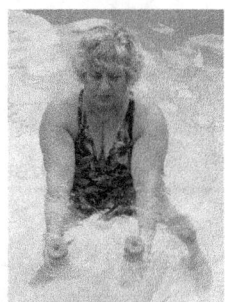

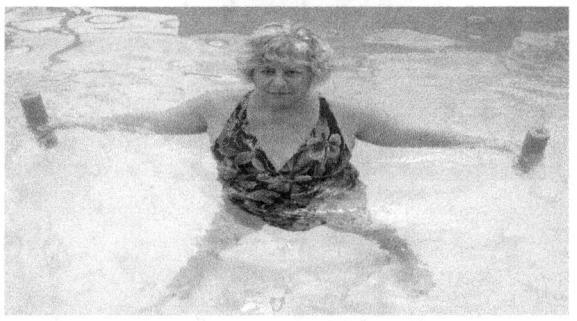

To Do: Place your hands on the center of the half noodle. Keep your feet flat on the bottom of the pool with your knees slightly bent. Inhale, and as you exhale bring the pool noodle toward the sides of your body. (Keep the noodle half way in the water). Inhale and as you exhale, bring the noodle back to the front of your chest. Repeat for a total of at least eight repetitions.

Arms and Shoulders

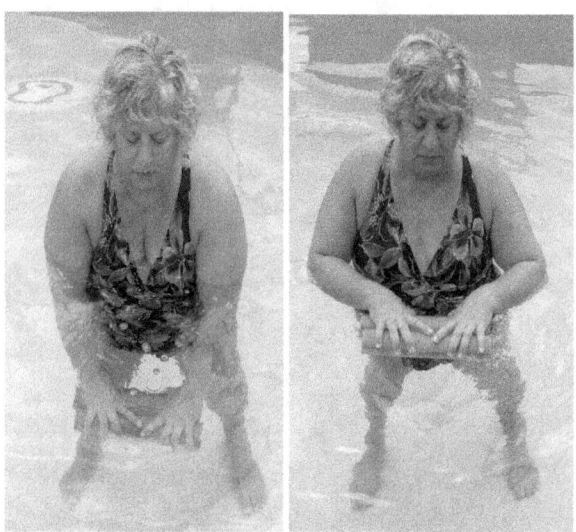

To Do: Place your hands on the center of both of the half noodles. Keep your feet flat on the bottom of the pool with your knees slightly bent. Inhale, and as you exhale bring the pool noodle toward the bottom of the pool right in front of your body. Inhale and as you exhale, bring the noodles back to the front of your chest at the top of the water. Repeat for a total of at least eight repetitions.

NOTE: You can keep the pool noodles under the water the whole time to make it easier on your shoulders.

Arms and Shoulders

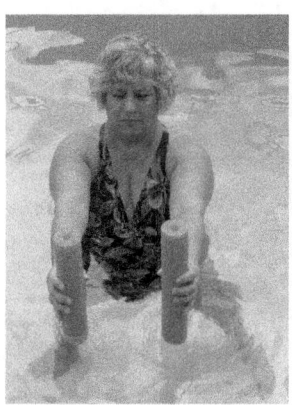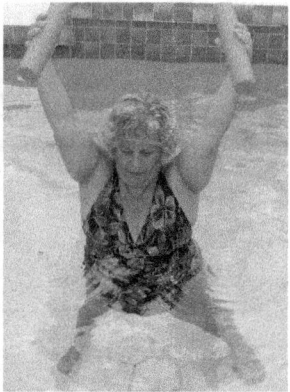

To Do: Place your hands on the center of the half noodle. Keep your feet flat on the bottom of the pool with your knees slightly bent. Inhale, and as you exhale bring the pool noodles straight up towards the sky right in front of your body.

Inhale and as you exhale, bring the noodle back to the front of your chest. Repeat for a total of at least eight repetitions.

Arms and Shoulders

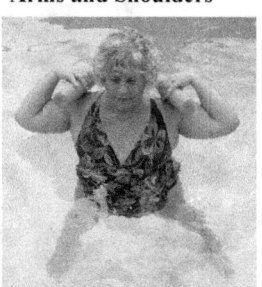

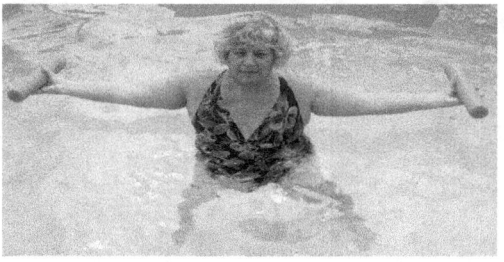

To Do: Place your hands on the center of the half noodle with your palms up. Your arms will be extended straight out by your side. Keep your feet flat on the bottom of the pool with your knees slightly bent. Inhale, and as you exhale bring the pool noodles toward your shoulders. Inhale and as you exhale, bring the noodles back out to the starting position. Repeat for a total of at least eight repetitions.

Arms and Shoulders

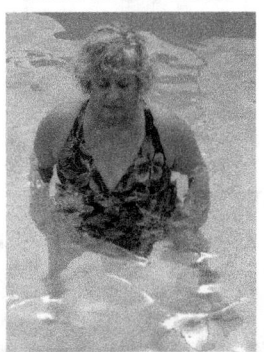

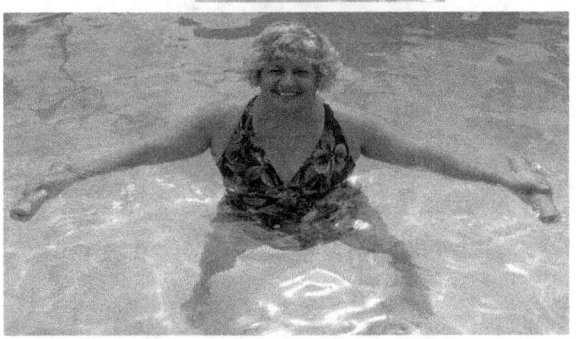

To Do: Place your hands on the center of the half noodle with the palms of your hand facing down. Keep your feet flat on the bottom of the pool with your knees slightly bent. Inhale, and as you exhale bring the noodles down toward the sides of your body. Inhale and as you exhale, bring the noodle back to the top of the water. Repeat for a total of at least eight repetitions.

Arms and Shoulders

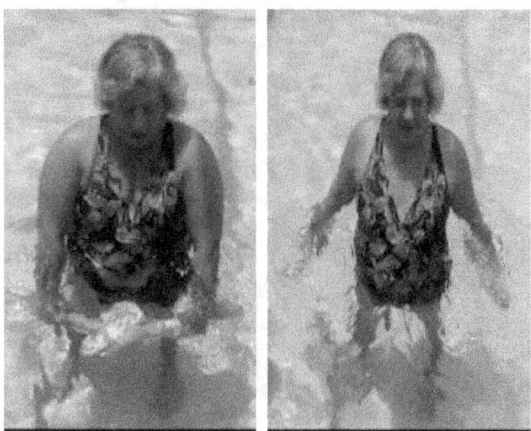

To Do: Place your hands on the center of the half noodle with the palms of your hand facing down. Keep your feet flat on the bottom of the pool with your knees slightly bent.

Your hands will be in front of your body-in the water with palms facing towards you. Inhale, and as you exhale bring the noodles out towards the sides of your body. Inhale and as you exhale, bring the noodle back to in front of your body. This is a nice and gentle shoulder rotation forward and backward.

Repeat for a total of at least eight repetitions.

Arms and Shoulders and Waistline

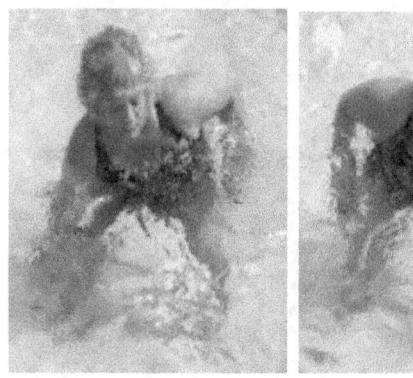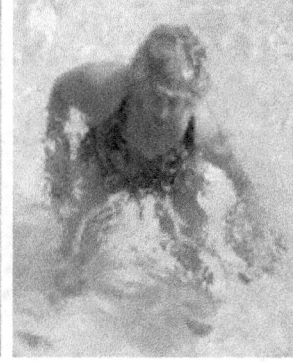

To Do: Place your hands on the center of the half noodle with the palms of your hand facing down. Keep your feet flat on the bottom of the pool with your knees slightly bent. Inhale, and as you exhale bring the noodle in your right hand down towards your right knee and return to center. Inhale and as you exhale, bring the noodle in your left hand down towards your left knee and return to center. Repeat for a total of at least eight repetitions on each side.

Waistline

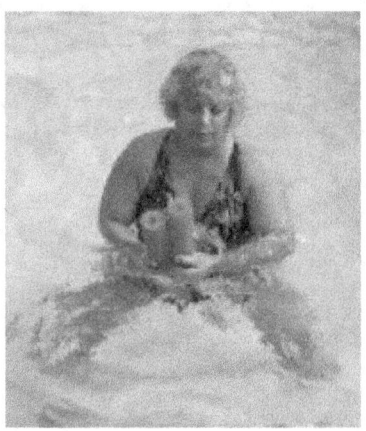

Starting Position

To Do: Place your hands on the center of the half noodle with the palms of your hand facing down. Keep your feet flat on the bottom of the pool with your knees slightly bent (you will be in a slight squatting position for this). Hold both noodles together in both of your hands and hold them halfway in the water.

Waistline

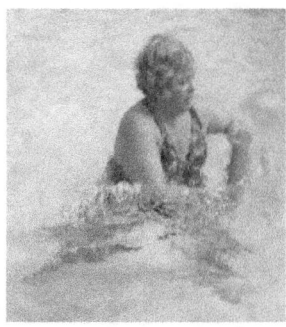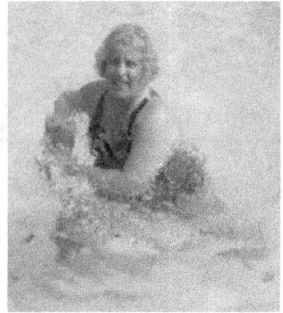

To Do: Begin in the starting position. Inhale, and as you exhale bring the noodles together towards the left sides of your body. Inhale and as you exhale, bring the noodle back to center (in front of your body). Inhale, and as you exhale bring the noodles together towards the right side of your body. Inhale and as you exhale, bring the noodle back to center (in front of your body). Repeat for a total of at least eight repetitions.

Waistline

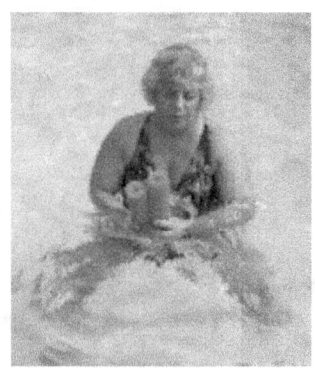

To Do: Place your hands on the center of the half noodle with the palms of your hand facing down. Keep your feet flat on the bottom of the pool with your knees slightly bent (you will be in a slight squatting position for this). Hold both noodles together in both of your hands and hold them halfway in the water.

Inhale and as you exhale bring both of the noodles down towards the inside of your legs as you round your back. Inhale and as you exhale, release back to starting positions. Do at least eight repetitions.

Waistline– Roll

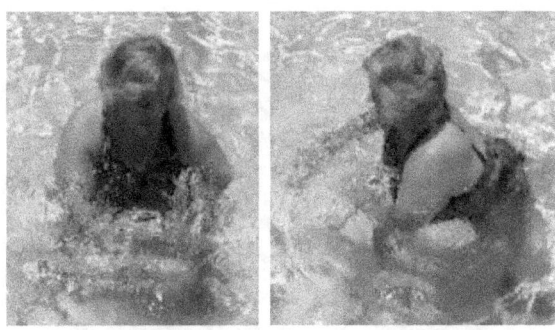

To Do: Place your hands on the center of the half noodle with the palms of your hand facing down. Keep your feet flat on the bottom of the pool with your knees slightly bent (you will be in a slight squatting position for this). Now begin rolling one hand over the other right in front of you. For variation, turn towards your right as you continue to rolls the pool noodles and then turn towards your left. Continue for at least eight repetitions on each side.

Triceps

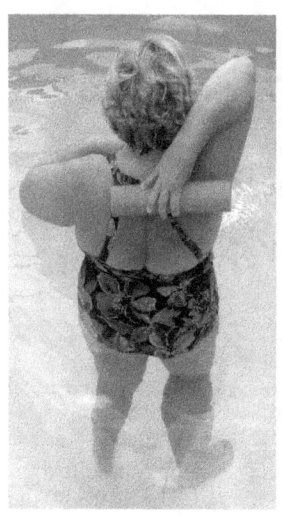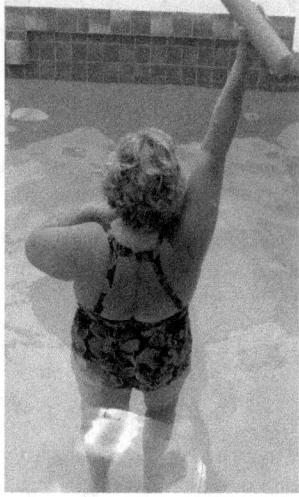

To Do: Stand with your feet shoulder width apart. Hold the pool noodle between your hands. Extend your right arm directly over your head (keep arm close to your right ear). Now, bend your right elbow and allow your hand with the noodle in it to rest on your back. Inhale, and as you exhale, lift your right arm straight overhead (as if you were going to through ball). Repeat for eight repetitions.

When finished, repeat this exercise using your left arm.

Triceps Variation

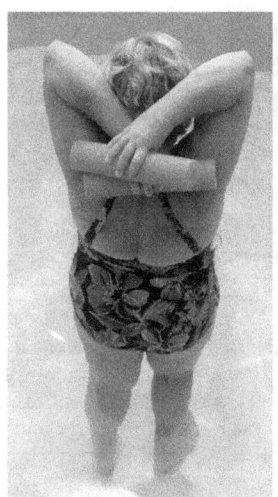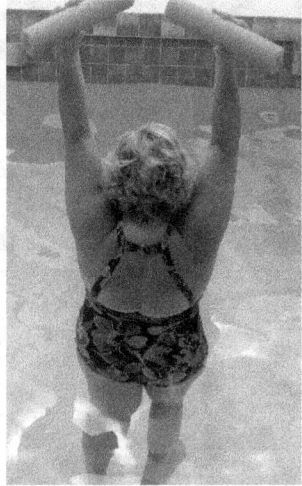

To Do: Stand with your feet shoulder width apart. Hold the pool noodles with your hands. Extend both of your arms directly over your head (keep arm close to your right ear). Now, bend both of your elbows at the same time and allow your hands with the noodle in them to rest on your back. Inhale, and as you exhale, lift your arms straight overhead (as if you were going to through ball). Repeat for eight repetitions.

Triceps

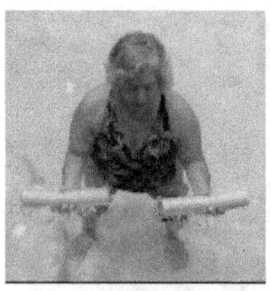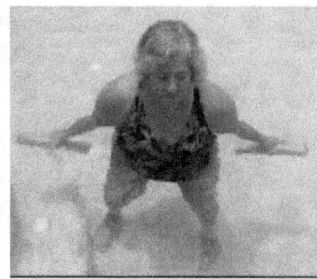

To Do: Stand with your feet shoulder width apart. Hold the pool noodles with your hands with your palms facing upward. Inhale and as you exhale, bring your arms straight back from your sides. Do NOT lean forward. Stand tall. Inhale again and you exhale, bring your arms straight out in front of you. Repeat for eight repetitions.

Back

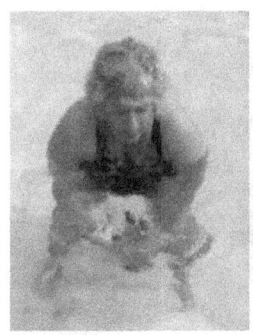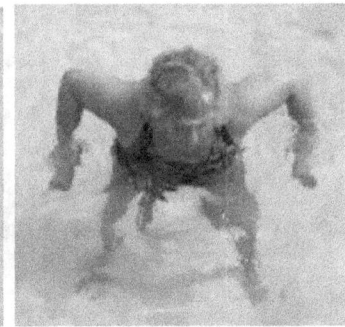

To Do: Stand with your feet shoulder width apart. Hold the pool noodles in the center with your hands. Bring both of the noodles together in front of you deep in the water. Round your back.

Inhale and as you exhale, bring your elbows straight up towards the sky. Inhale again and as you exhale, return your hands back down into the water directly in front of your body. Your back should NOT move at all during this exercise. Repeat for eight repetitions.

Basic Water Moves

Knee-ups

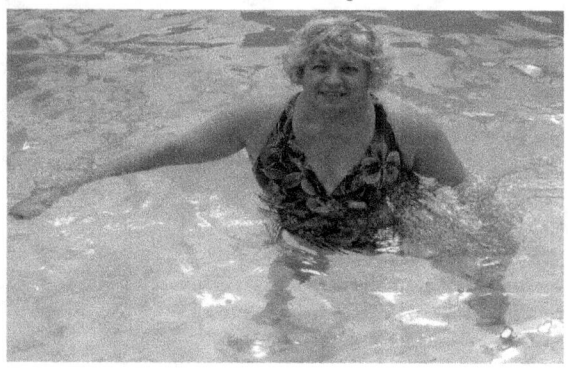

Level One -Single Knee Lifts-Lift your right knee up toward the right side of your body and bring your right hand with the pool noodle in it down to touch the right knee. Return the right foot back down to the bottom of the pool and straighten up your body. Do eight repetitions on the right. Repeat on the left side of the body by bringing left knee and left hand together.

Level Two -Alternating Knee Lifts -Alternate lifting the right and left knees. Touch the right hand to the left knee and the left hand to the right knee. Work up to 25 repetitions.

Level Three -Alternating Knee Lifts –Add speed and movements to this exercise. You can also move forward and backward while doing this exercise and in a right/left circle.

Front Leg Lifts

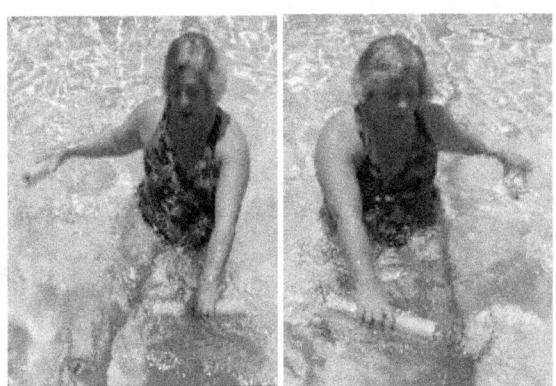

Level One-Begin with both feet planted firmly on the bottom of the pool and with your knees soft. Now, inhale and bring your left leg straight up in front of you as high as you comfortably can, hold for a few seconds, and then as exhale, bring your leg back down to the starting position. You can try to touch your foot to the ball. Do a total of eight repetitions and then repeat exercise on the other leg.

Level Two- Alternate lifting your right and left leg. Continue alternative the front leg lifts for a total of 16 repetitions.

Level Three- Add speed, hopping from right to left leg. Move forward and backward while alternating front leg lifts.

Side Leg Lifts

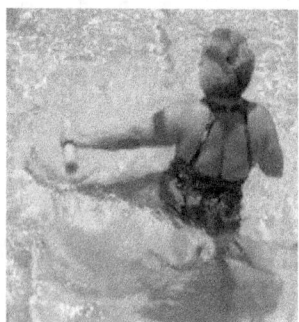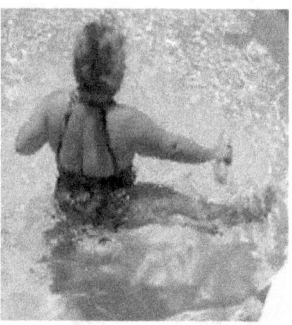

Level One-Inhale and as you exhale lift your right leg straight up at your side as high as you comfortably can. Inhale and as you exhale bring the leg back to the bottom of the pool. Repeat for a total of eight repetitions. Repeat the entire exercise on your left leg.

Level Two-Lift your right leg up to your right side and return to the starting position. Then, lift your left leg up to your left side and return to the starting position. Repeat alternating between the right leg and the left leg for 16 repetitions.

Level Three-Add speed to the exercise shifting rapidly between the right and left leg lifts. Move forward and backward and even sideways from one end of the pool to the other. You can vary your speed and even add a double hop on one foot to add variety to your workout.

Inside Leg Lifts

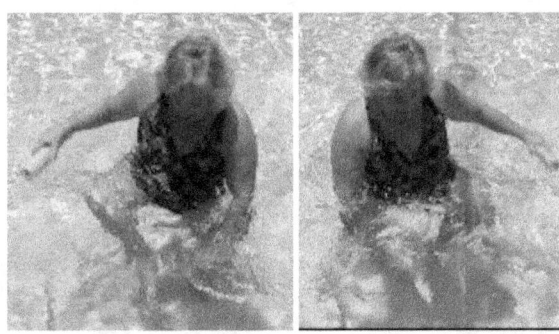

Level One-Inhale and as you exhale lift your right leg straight up in front of you as high as you comfortably can. Inhale and as you exhale bring the leg back to the bottom of the pool. Repeat for a total of eight repetitions. Repeat the entire exercise on your left leg.

Level Two-Lift your right leg up in front of you and return to the starting position. Then, lift your left leg up in front of you and return to the starting position. Repeat alternating between the right leg and the left leg for a total of 16 repetitions.

Level Three-Add speed to the exercise shifting rapidly between the right and left leg lifts. You can also move forward and backward as you do this exercise. You can vary your speed and even add a double hop on one foot to add variety to your workout.

Kick-Backs

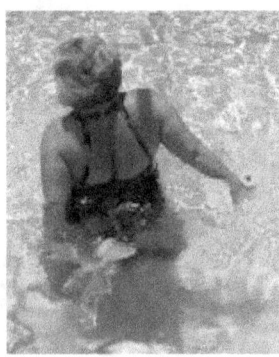 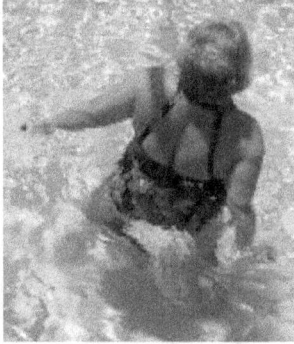

Level One-Lift your right leg straight up in back of you as high as you comfortably can. Inhale and as you exhale bring the leg back to the bottom of the pool. Repeat for a total of eight repetitions. Repeat the entire exercise on your left leg.

Level Two-Lift your right leg up in front of you and return to the starting position. Then, lift your left leg up in back of you and return to the starting position. Repeat alternating between the right leg and the left leg for a total of 16 repetitions.

Level Three-Add speed to the exercise shifting rapidly between the right and left leg lifts. You can move forward and backward and vary your speed. Add a double hop on one foot to add variety to your workout.

Kick-Backs (2)

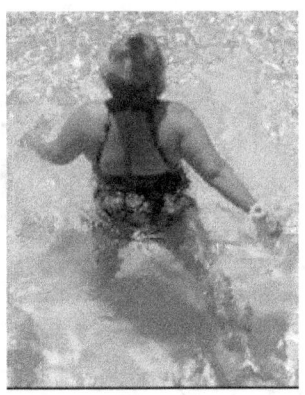

Level One- Lift your right leg straight up in behind you. Inhale and as you exhale bring the leg back to the bottom of the pool. Repeat for a total of eight repetitions. Repeat the entire exercise on your left leg.

Level Two-Lift your right leg up behind you and return to the starting position. Then, lift your left leg up behind you and return to the starting position. Repeat alternating between lifting the right and left leg behind you for 16 repetitions.

Level Three-Add speed to the exercise shifting rapidly between the right and left leg lifts. Move forward and backward as you do this exercise.

Stretches

1. Shoulder Stretch

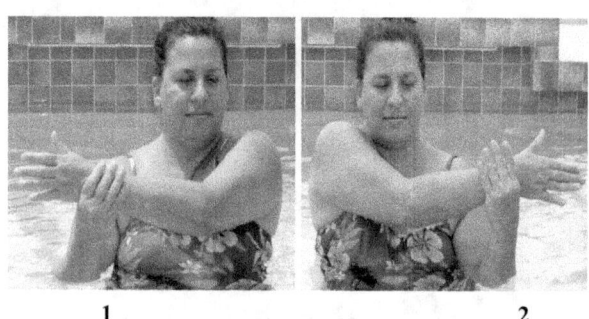

1   2

To Do: Begin the cool down by bring your straight left arm across the front of your body and gently grasp your left wrist with your right hand (as shown in picture #1). Gently press the left arm toward your right arm.

Be sure to keep your hips and body straight and looking forward. Do not force the stretch and be sure to inhale and exhale freely and easily. Release the arm.

Now, take your straight right arm and bring it across the front of your body and gently grasp your right wrist with your left hand and press the arms towards your left arm (as shown in picture #2). Release the arm. Repeat on both sides for an additional two more times.

2. Shoulder Hug

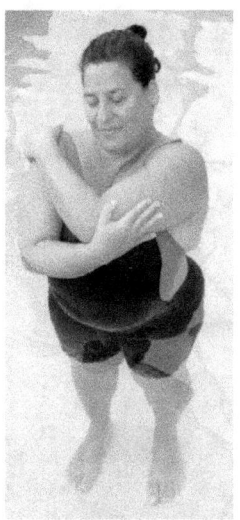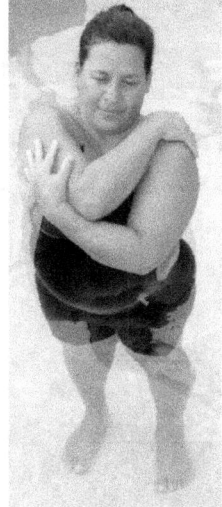

To Do: A great shoulder stretch in the 'hug'. Just wrap your arms around each other and give yourself a big hug. Inhale and exhale freely and easily.

Release your hug and switch your arms around and give yourself another big hug. Inhale and exhale freely and easily. Repeat the hug for an additional two more times on each side.

Stretch

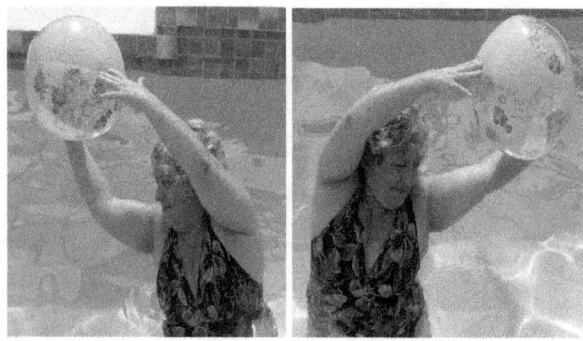

To Do: Begin this exercise by standing with feet flat on the bottom of the pool and shoulder width apart. Inhale and reach your arms straight upward from your body while holding the ball between your hands. Exhale and bring arms to one side of the body.

Inhale and as you exhale return to the starting position. Repeat on the other side. Perform this stretch a total of eight times on each side.

Hip Stretch

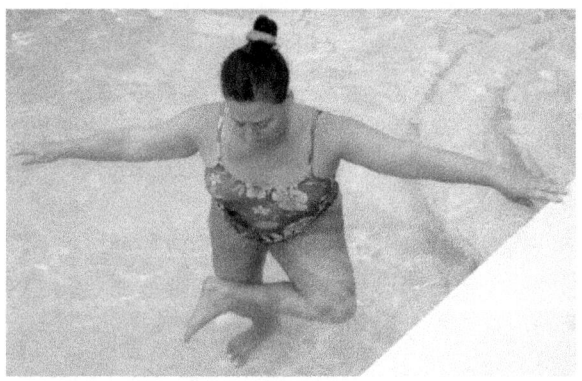

To Do: Stand with both of your feet planted firmly on the bottom of the pool shoulder width apart. Bend your left knee and bring your left up the front of your body and place it just above your knee.

Now, as you exhale, slowly bend your right knee and allow yourself to sink into the water as far as you can comfortably go. Hold, and then release into starting position. Repeat this exercise on the other side using your right foot on your left thigh.

To add more depth to this hip stretch exercise you can do the following: As you sink into the water as far down as you can go, hold that position and lift up off the heel of your foot.

Cool Down

Cool Downs are a series of movements that are used after an exercise class as a means to return the heart rate back to its normal pre-exercise rate. The more you exercise, the stronger your heart and lungs will become and the shorter the period of time it will take for the heart rate to return to normal. If you need help in adapting any of these exercises to your own specific limitations, just drop me an email at RevReikiND@cs.com and we can discuss options.

Cool Down

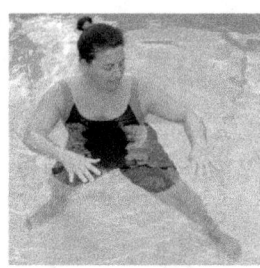 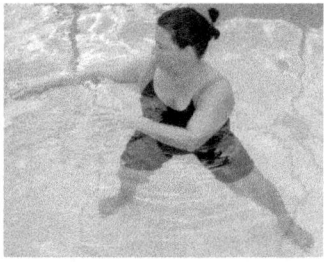

To Do: You can add mindfulness and breath to this cool down exercise. To do this exercise, spread your legs apart as far as you comfortably can to maintain your body's balance in the water.

Place your hands, palm down, at the very top of the water and pretend that there are flower petals floating on the top of the water. Gently push the flower petals to the left and then to right trying not to disturb the petals, or the water.

About the Author

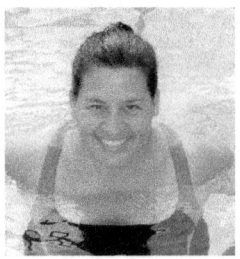

Francine Milford, LMT, CTN, has had a very long career in the Fitness Industry. Working for more than 25 years in a variety of sports and exercise related classes, she is also an avid walker and enjoys reading a book audio tape while bicycling around the neighborhood.

A national and state licensed massage therapist and personal trainer, Francine has achieved certifications through the YMCA S.A.F.E. Aerobic Program, AEA Aquatics Exercise Association, ESA Exercise Safety Association, and AFAA Aerobics Fitness Association. She has also received the Tai Chi for Arthritis Certification having studied under Dr. Paul Lam, as well as, 180 hours of professional training in Tai Kwan Do. She has taught such classes as Kick Boxing, Bench Stepping, Low Impact Aerobics, High Impact Aerobics, Basic Floor and Senior Aerobics and all types of Water Aerobic classes.

As a fitness specialist, Francine has been hired to lead classes and workshops at offices, condo organizations, clubs and private groups. Having spent the last 20 years working with the senior population, Francine has developed exercises that are both safe and effective for those with physical limitations. Visit online at www.H2OWorkouts.com or at www.ReikiCenterofVenice.com

www.ingramcontent.com/pod-product-compliance
Lightning Source LLC
Chambersburg PA
CBHW071248280526
45788CB00004B/1627